ELLEN SHULER

THRIVING WITHOUT SUGAR

A Pocket Guide to Leaving the Cravings Behind and Taking Back Your Vibrancy

First edition

This book was professionally typeset on Reedsy.
Find out more at reedsy.com

He who has his health has every dream. He
who does not have his health has only one

- ANON

Contents

1

INTRODUCTION

How bad could sugar be? I mean everybody eats it. Even the girl scouts sell it! Well, it turns out very bad in high quantities, and because of its addictive quality, almost everybody who eats ANY sugar eats too much sugar.

Too much sugar effects your mood, your energy, your bone health, your liver, your kidneys, your brain, your heart, your teeth, and puts you at risk for diabetes and cancer. It can also make you gain weight. Rather than try to figure out exactly how much sugar is "safe", it's much easier to remove it from your diet altogether.

The majority of people have a sweet tooth, but I'm living proof that once you give up sugar completely, even for a relatively short period of time, you won't even think about it anymore. It's similar to the difference between a heroin addict and the person who has never done heroin. The person who has never done heroin never even thinks about what he's missing. Addiction to sugar has been compared to the addiction related to alcohol and morphine like drugs. Take heart, though, if my body and mind can break the addiction to sugar, anybody's can.

My Story

When I was in my late 30's I seemed perfectly healthy. I was the right weight. I had good muscle tone. I didn't take any medication. Blood pressure low. Cholesterol low. Strong heartbeat. I was slender and athletic in build. I was the right weight and I worked out every weekend and swam during the week. Who could be healthier? At least that's what I thought!

Despite all of this, I had a strange intangible, growing malaise. I was cold all the time. I wasn't happy very much. My eyes watered incessantly. I had strange aches and pains. it was nothing that would bring me down and put me in bed for a couple of days, but it just was just a malingering sort of unhappiness and weakness. I was tired a lot. I felt something must be WRONG. I seemed to have lost my vibrancy.

Fortunately, I was working for the IT department of a large hospital and had really good health insurance, even if Western medicine was all it covered. I paraded around to the thyroid Doctor, the hormone Doctor, the rheumatologist - everybody you could think of. I remember those first visits when they would say, "Okay! let's run a bunch of tests and we'll get to the bottom of this." I would leave the office so happy - so optimistic that finally we were going to get to the bottom of this and figure out what was wrong with me. Then it would be time for that second visit. They would have all the test results in hand. I could see on their faces that this was going to be another one of those crushing second office visits.

"Well, everything seems to be in normal range" they would say. While that made me happy that everything was in normal range, I was once again left with no answers, wondering "Where do I go from here?" And so it would go. Doctor after doctor after doctor. I started to fear I was looking like a hypochondriac.

I didn't see that anything was really seriously wrong with me. Nothing was bleeding. nothing was knocking me down and keeping me from work. But boy I sure dragged through life. As far as my digestive system went, well, that movement most people do daily I only did weekly. This went on for years. It's a wonder I didn't contract colon cancer. The only time things would move for me was on the weekends when I would work out for a couple hours at a time. Again, I thought I was in good health I was the right weight and my skin look reasonably good and clear so what could possibly be wrong with me?

Just before I turned 40, it was recommended that I go on an anti-candida diet. Nothing that feeds the candida in the stomach. I decided to try it.

I had gotten to the point where whenever I ate something, I felt bad afterwards. I have every reason to think that this was from a bad habit I had adopted of taking ibuprofen on an empty stomach. I did this to battle the strange joint pains I had. I didn't realize that this could lead to leaky gut syndrome. I think that's the reason that every time I ate something I felt so bad afterwards.

I remember the first day of my diet in fall of my 39th year. That day my large IT department of about 125 people which spanned an entire floor in a large office building held a holiday potluck. There were all kinds of dishes but I was serious about starting this diet so I only ate the steamed vegetable dishes or the raw vegetable dishes. To my amazement a half hour later my stomach felt GOOD instead of bad.

I remember how elated I felt that day. I was so desperate that it seemed like sticking to the diet was simple. I ate animal protein and steamed vegetables for the most part and when I say vegetables I don't mean the starchy kind. I stuck with cauliflower, broccoli, celery, carrots, cabbage, kale and some very clean salads. No salad dressing. Just lemon and sometimes olive oil.

After about 2 months of that I started to feel better. I made a list of over 20 things that had improved in my life, such as my digestive system working normally. No more gas. Mood swings went away. I cried less. I was more optimistic. I didn't seem to have allergies anymore.

It was about then that the "Aha!" moment came to me as to just how much power I had over my health by simply controlling my diet. I began to see food in a different way. When I walked by a vending machine, I saw almost nothing in that box as food. I saw all of it as overhead to my body that my body would have to digest but would get nothing good out of.

After six months on the diet, I backed off and became much less strict. Despite going off the strict diet after only six months, I didn't so much as come down with sniffles for 4 FULL YEARS! My allergies to plants went away, and have not come back despite the fact it's been over 10 years. If this can happen for me, imagine what can happen for you!

2

THE DEMON SUGAR

I'm not going to go into depth regarding the evils of sugar. If you've made it to this book, I'm guessing you already know that you would be improving your health and your chance of avoiding certain diseases by giving up sugar. Still, it will be good motivation to review some of these diseases that sugar is involved with.

Cancer

It's been said that sugar is the food of choice of cancerous tumors. According to doctors, "Human epidemiologic studies and mechanistic preclinical studies in multiple cancers support a causal link between excess sugar and cancer." (Epner, M., Yang, P., Wagner, R. W., & Cohen, L. (2022). Understanding the Link between Sugar and Cancer: An Examination of the Preclinical and Clinical Evidence. *Cancers, 14*(24), 6042.) Causal link! That means they are saying sugar causes cancer, and since they use dyed sugar water in PET scans to detect cancerous tumors, I think we can all do that math. Cancer likes sugar! It's been said that nothing tastes as good as being thin feels. I would go one step further and say that nothing tastes as good as being cancer free feels!

Diabetes

Diabetes runs in my family, and I have long believed that I am pre-diabetic. It was easy to see how much of my malaise was cleared up with giving up sugar back in my late 30's, and I seem to have a weakness for sugar. I do much better on a low carbohydrate diet, and my blood sugar seems to be much more stable with a diet rich in animal protein and non-starchy vegetables.

When searching the internet, I notice that there seems to be a bit of resistance as to naming sugar the main culprit for the meteoric rise of Diabetes in our country. However, one must be aware of sugar cane growers and food producers who make lots of money producing sugary foods. I think enough medical professionals and scientists have weighed in on the subject that I don't need to emphasize the relationship sugar has in causing diabetes. According to the CDC, 38 million people in the United States have diabetes and 98 million adults have pre-diabetes. That means that more than 130 million people in a country of about 330 million are affected by diabetes in some way, or 39% of the population!

The good news is that a lot of times diabetes can be avoided through lifestyle changes, the most important of which is diet.

Obesity

Dr. Robert Lustig is an author and renowned doctor who has published a book called "Fat Chance." Dr. Lustig mentions in his book that he is a childhood obesity doctor, a practice that didn't even exist a few decades ago. In his book he details many evils of sugar, and if you are in need of motivation, I strongly suggest you get a copy of that book. One of my favorite stories in that book is the story of leptin and sugar. Leptin is the hormone that tells your body it's full, and that you can burn more calories. Leptin therefore helps your body maintain a normal weight on a long-term basis. In the mid 1970's, they isolated leptin and figured they would mass produce it, and obesity would be a thing of the past! Great idea, except, it turns out, sugar numbs the receptor that "listens" for leptin. So apparently, leptin won't help you feel "full" if you eat enough sugar to deaden your body's receptor to leptin!

Osteoporosis:

According to some metabolism doctors, "…sugar may lead to osteoporosis by increasing inflammation, hyperinsulinemia, increased renal acid load, reduced calcium intake, and increased urinary calcium excretion." (DiNicolantonio, J. J., Mehta, V., Zaman, S. B., & O'Keefe, J. H. (2018, June 1). *Not salt but sugar as an etiological in Osteoporosis: a review.*) In other words, sugar prevents your body from absorbing as much calcium, and if you are peeing out more calcium, where could that calcium be coming from? I'm guessing the bones. By the way, hyperinsulinemia is an increased level of insulin, which as you have probably heard, is a big factor in diabetes.

Heart Disease

According to Harvard Medical School, sugar can have a significant impact on your heart. "Over the course of the 15-year study, people who got 17% to 21% of their calories from added sugar had a 38% higher risk of dying from cardiovascular disease compared with those who consumed 8% of their calories as added sugar." (Harvard Health. (2022, January 6). *The sweet danger of sugar.*) I don't even think I want the risk to my heart that comes from only 8% of my calories coming from added sugar, thank you!

Other health issues

I'm sure you are aware of other health problems with sugar intake. Not to mention the battle of the bulge and tooth decay. If you're anything like me, the more sugar you get the more sugar you want. We'll explore the addictive nature of sugar in the next chapter.

3

WHY SUGAR IS SO ADDICTIVE

If you think sugar is just a habit, and doesn't have physiological implications of addiction, think again. Doctors who published an article in an international journal on nutrition, diet and the nervous system did a very interesting study involving rats. They measured such things as circadian rhythm, body temperature and behavioral changes. They concluded that the effects of sugar addiction, withdrawal and relapse were similar to those found in drugs that are normally abused and thought to have addictive qualities.

Sugar stimulates pleasure centers in the brain. Mount Sinai Health Systems concluded that consumption of sugar results in neurochemical changes in the brain and is therefore expected to have addictive potential. Sound familiar? I hear those words a lot when heroin is talked about. I know friends who try to "cut down" on their sugar intake, and I rarely hear of success regarding their endeavor. I liken it to trying to reduce heroin intake. I doubt that has much success, either.

Candida and Sugar

Candida is a yeast that naturally occurs in the body and the gut. According to physician Amy Myers, and many other sources, yeast feeds on sugar. While the existence of candida in the gut is normal, an overgrowth is not. Normally the good bacteria that live in our gut keep the candida in check, but an overgrowth in candida overwhelms the good bacteria. When that happens, it's easy to see how the gut biome then contributes to more sugar cravings, since the candida that live in the gut now outnumber the good bacteria, and they love sugar. When giving up sugar, I picture myself starving the candida in my gut. It helps me during the hard times.

Lastly, there is the social aspect of giving up sugar. Besides having to pass on dessert, giving up sugar means giving up alcohol. Don't worry, though. I cover tricks and tips regarding this in the next section.

4

LEAVING SUGAR BEHIND

When it comes to giving up sugar, I want to tell you that I've never found anybody weaker toward sugar than I am when I'm in the throes. When I have successfully given up sugar, I feel strong and free from temptation. It's an amazing shift. If I can do that, anybody can.

So now, I invite you to begin leaving sugar behind. You have the energy and momentum right now, as you've read this far. There is no shortcut. If you have ideas about "quitting slowly", I urge you to reconsider. Let me introduce you to a powerful tool I learned a few years ago.

The 15 Twinkie theory of change

I was studying under a life coach named Bill Sumner, of the Inevitable You a few years ago.

What he shared was a radical theory, but he backed it up with data from heart doctors who had patients that were on a lifestyle road toward serious heart disease or worse. Here's how the 15 twinkie theory of change goes.

Imagine that you've been eating 15 twinkies a day for as long as you can remember, and now you're being told that you will have serious health consequences if you don't give up ALL twinkies. So, you figure that you'll give up one twinkie every week, and in 15 weeks, you'll be completely off of your twinkie habit.

Week one is tough. You aren't thinking about the 14 twinkies you GET to have, but instead are thinking about the 1 twinkie you DON'T get to have. It's so HARD to be without that 15th twinkie you are used to! Week two, is even worse as you have TWO twinkies you can't have every day.

At the end of week two, what happens? Your best friend has a birthday party and you are, of course invited. You HAVE to attend. She's your best friend. And what is she serving at the party? FRIED TWINKIES! OMG! You go to the party. You eat so many fried twinkies you get sick. The next day your feel so sick, guilty and discouraged, that you scrap the whole thing and give up trying to change!

Now, compare that scenario to the one that follows.

Week one, you give up ALL 15 twinkies. Day one is REALLY hard. So is day two. So is the whole week, really. But by the end of week one, you're feeling pretty strong and proud of yourself. You're seeing a difference on the scale, and that's really building your confidence. You feel a strength that comes from discipline. And all those walks you had to take to get your mind off of twinkies have started to become pretty enjoyable. Week two, while still tough, isn't near as hard as week one was.

Now here comes your friend's birthday party at the end of week two. You still go to the party. When the twinkies come around, you find that your cravings have eased somewhat. Oh, you still have a twinkie, or maybe even two. But the next morning, you don't feel near as bad as you would have felt if you had binged! The scale still shows progress, and you realize how far you've come in just a couple of weeks, and you jump right back on your program of twinkie abstinence.

Lots of data, especially among heart patients, supports this style of change. I know for me, giving up sugar must be done cold turkey, and I look forward to the freedom and strength I feel in a few days.

PREPARING TO GIVING UP SUGAR

Okay it's time to get started but here's a couple of things before we do.

First of all, get all the sugar and bread and flour and cereal out of your house. Temptation and easy accessibility will not help you. If you can't get it out of your house and throw it away then box it up, tape it up and put the box somewhere where you won't think about it.

Second, realize that this is going to be a fight. The natural cravings and the Candida in your gut are not going to go down easily. Before you start make a list of 5 to 10 times in your life that you have had a victory. It doesn't matter if it's a small victory or a large victory. Write down these victories and leave space between them. The space is so that over the next few days you can elaborate on those victories, and talk about how empowered you felt after these victories. Keep this list vary accessible, so you can whip it out when you feel discouraged or weak.

Third, it helps me to do an intermittent fast before I give up sugar, or start any new eating habit. Anytime I fast, I feel that my body gets back into balance, and begins to crave the foods that are good for it, such as animal protein and vegetables. There are tons of resources about intermittent fasting easily available in books and on the internet, so I'm not going to go into it here.

When the going gets tough, keep the following in mind. You're most likely going to get down or depressed. Know that these feelings are natural because your blood sugar has a lot to do with your mood. When these times come think about how wonderful it's going to be to have clearer skin, better energy, better stamina, a healthy body and a calm, strong mind. And don't forget to review your victories list.

The Rules

Sugar is tough to give up, and you have to give up so many foods that it's easier to talk about what your diet WILL include than what it won't. This is only MY list, and if you see any problem with giving up any of these foods, you should consult your doctor.

The following foods are ILLEGAL!

- **Sugar and sugar substitutes in all form** – Sugar substitutes and artificial sugars keep your body craving sweets, and we want to kill those cravings as quickly as possible. No sweets, candy, or desserts period! No sweetened drinks.
- **Flour and grains** – It's impossible to eat bread or flour without

sugar, so just skip it. Also, grains tend to raise your blood sugar, and we want to avoid those spikes. No cereals with any sugar in their ingredients, which is most if not all of them. If you want to eat a sweet potato without any sugar on it, that's fine. Also, putting butter and cinnamon on the sweet potato is fine, as the cinnamon helps to regulate blood sugar. A little brown rice is OK on occasion.

- **Alcohol** – Well, you knew this was coming. Alcohol tends to throw off blood sugar levels, and turns to sugar in the body. Avoid it.
- **Fruits** (except lemons and limes)– In the beginning, it's best to keep yourself from running to fruit to get the sugar your body craves. After you've gone a couple weeks or so, it's recommended that you introduce low sugar fruits back into your diet if you need to, such as berries. Lemon and Lime are always OK. Fruit juice is off the table. All that sugar without the fiber to slow absorption of sugar is a no-no.
- **Processed foods with sugar** – Beware of things like salad dressing. I squeeze juice from a fresh lemon onto salad, and maybe just a little avocado oil. When you give up sugar, you'll find that you taste "real food" so much more, and don't need to use things like salad dressing so much. Soups will tend to have sugar in them as well and should probably be avoided when in doubt.

So, what's left?

Here's the diet that was probably intended for you and I all along, but certain stick to it when you give up sugar.

<u>The following foods are LEGAL!</u>

- **Animal Protein**
- **Healthy fat sources** – eggs, avocados and avocado oil, nuts, seeds, olive oil, coconut oil, unsweetened yogurt.
- **Vegetables** – broccoli, cauliflower, carrots, celery, salads dressed with lemon and/or non-seed- based oil, asparagus, zucchini.
- **Complex Carbohydrates** – beans, sweet potatoes, butternut squash, spaghetti squash, brown rice.
- **Unsweetened beverages** – water, sparkling water, unsweetened coffee, tea.

Helpful Tips

Here's a few helpful tips that have really helped me get through the first few days, and find the strength and pride to fuel the journey through being independent of sugar cravings

Squeeze Lemon or Lime in your water

This helps to feel like you're drinking something a little more special than water. Also, lemons and limes are both rich in nutrients, and we want your body to go back to craving the nutrients it was born to use.

Order Club Soda with Lime When You're at Social Events

This will keep you away from alcohol, and you won't feel awkward not having a drink in your hands.

When feeling tempted, get some exercise

Take a walk. Go for a run. Get your adrenaline moving. This will get your adrenaline going and take your mind off of things.

Other Tricks

For the first few days, I like to mix up some unsweetened Greek yogurt, and enough cinnamon to make it look like chocolate pudding. This looks like a treat, but doesn't really taste like one. Still, the act of eating something creamy helps me feel like I'm treating myself, and cinnamon is great for normalizing blood sugar. After a couple days of this, I rarely need to go any farther with it, but it helps during those first couple of days.

5

YOUR WELL-DESERVED REWARDS

On the other side of the fight awaits amazing rewards. You will feel healthy and vibrant like you never have before.

There are a multitude of benefits that come from a diet free from sugar. I have listed them here but there are probably more:

- **It will be easier for you to reach your weight loss goals**
- **You will decrease your risk of getting diabetes, or be able to reduce your symptoms**
- **Your skin's aging process will slow**
- **Your immune system will improve and you will be less likely to get sick**
- **Your sugar cravings will be reduced or eliminated altogether**
- **Improved psychological health with less depression**
- **Your hunger will decrease**
- **You'll have more energy**
- **Your heart and brain will be healthier**

- **You will get fewer cavities**
- **General vibrancy**

I can attest to almost all of these being true. They have all come true for me whenever I've given up sugar.

Don't stop until you get there. Your health is worth every hardship that giving up sugar can throw at you. Remember; "He who has health has every dream, while he who has lost his health has only one dream." – Anon

I wish you the best of journeys, and good health for life! If you found this book helpful, I would be very appreciative if you left a favorable review on Amazon!

6

REFERENCES

Epner, M., Yang, P., Wagner, R. W., & Cohen, L. (2022). Understanding the Link between Sugar and Cancer: An Examination of the Preclinical and Clinical Evidence. *Cancers,* *14*(24), 6042. https://doi.org/10.3390/cancers14246042

A report card: Diabetes in the United States infographic. (2024, May 15). Diabetes. https://www.cdc.gov/diabetes/communication-resources/diabetes-statistics.html

(Amazon.com: Fat Chance: Beating the Odds Against Sugar, Processed Food, Obesity, and Disease (Audible Audio Edition): Robert H. Lustig, Jonathan Todd Ross, Penguin Audio: Books, n.d.)

Professional, C. C. M. (2024, May 1). *Leptin & Leptin Resistance.* Cleveland Clinic. https://my.clevelandclinic.org/health/articles/22446-leptin

DiNicolantonio, J. J., Mehta, V., Zaman, S. B., & O'Keefe, J. H. (2018, June

1). *Not salt but sugar as aetiological in Osteoporosis: a review.* https://pmc.ncbi.nlm.nih.gov/articles/PMC6140170/

Harvard Health. (2022, January 6). *The sweet danger of sugar.* https://www.health.harvard.edu/heart-health/the-sweet-danger-of-sugar

Wideman, C. H., Nadzam, G. R., & Murphy, H. M. (2005). Implications of an animal model of sugar addiction, withdrawal and relapse for human health. *Nutritional Neuroscience, 8*(5–6), 269–276. https://doi.org/10.1080/10284150500485221

"Sugar Addiction is Real – Here's What's Behind the Science and How to Quit" - Abby Haglage | Mount Sinai - New York. (n.d.). Mount Sinai Health System. https://www.mountsinai.org/about/newsroom/2019/sugar-addiction-is-real-heres-whats-behind-the-science-and-how-to-quit-abby-haglage

Myers, A. (2023, May 17). *9 foods to avoid if you have Candida.* Amy Myers MD. https://www.amymyersmd.com/blogs/articles/avoid-foods-candida

Sumner, W. (2020, December 7). *Why going "cold turkey" works better than an incremental approach to change - Inevitable You.* Inevitable You. https://inevitableyou.com/going-cold-turkey-works-better-than-incremental-approach-change/

Rd, R. a. M. (2024, June 25). *How cinnamon lowers blood sugar and helps diabetes.* Healthline. https://www.healthline.com/nutrition/cinnamon-and-diabetes

Rd, C. W. P. (2024, November 19). What happens to your body when you cut out sugar. *EatingWell.* https://www.eatingwell.com/article/7869775/what-happens-to-your-body-when-you-cut-out-sugar/

www.ingramcontent.com/pod-product-compliance
Lightning Source LLC
Chambersburg PA
CBHW072345270726
48659CB00023B/2395